Low Impact Exercises for Seniors

Energize Your Body, Empower Your Health, and Embrace Active Aging"

AGO XABARA

TABLE OF CONTENTS

INTRODUCTION

Dear Readers,

We are delighted to welcome you to this comprehensive guide designed specifically for seniors who are eager to embrace the benefits of exercise in a gentle and effective way. Aging should never be a barrier to maintaining a healthy and active lifestyle, and this book is here to guide you through a fulfilling fitness journey tailored to your needs.

In the pages that follow, you will discover a wealth of knowledge about low impact exercises carefully curated to enhance your strength, balance, flexibility, and overall well-being. Whether you are a seasoned fitness enthusiast or just starting out, our aim is to provide you with a supportive roadmap, ensuring that your fitness routine is not only enjoyable but also safe and beneficial.

We understand that each individual's fitness journey is unique, and that's why we have included a variety of exercises catering to different levels of mobility and health conditions. From seated cardio workouts and gentle yoga stretches to mindfulness practices and motivational tips, this book covers a wide spectrum of activities to cater to your specific needs and preferences.

Remember, this journey is not just about physical well-being—it's also about embracing a positive mindset, fostering connections, and finding joy in every movement. We encourage you to approach these exercises with enthusiasm, curiosity, and a sense of accomplishment. Together, let's embark on a path to better health, increased vitality, and a happier, more active lifestyle.

Thank you for choosing "Low Impact Exercises for Seniors." We believe in your potential, and we're here to support you every step of the way.

Wishing you a fulfilling and energizing fitness journey ahead!

Warmest regards,

CHAPTER ONE

UNDERSTANDING THE IMPORTANCE OF EXERCISE FOR SENIORS

Benefits of Exercise for Older Adults

Certainly! For older persons, regular exercise has a wealth of advantages that may considerably improve their general quality of life.

1.Improved Physical Health:

Regular physical exercise lowers the risk of chronic illnesses including heart disease, diabetes, and osteoporosis in older persons and helps them maintain a healthy weight. Additionally, exercise promotes improved circulation, which may reduce the risk of stroke and enhance general cardiovascular health.

2. Increased Flexibility and Mobility:

Exercise may increase mobility and lower the risk of falling, particularly when it focuses on flexibility and balance. This is crucial for senior people since falls may result in significant injury. Strengthening exercises also encourage improved posture and facilitate everyday tasks.

3. Increased Bone Density and Muscle Strength:

Exercises that increase muscular strength and muscle mass in older persons are known as strength training. This is essential for avoiding weakness and supporting joints. Exercises that include lifting weights also increase bone density, which lowers the risk of fractures and osteoporosis.

4. Pain Management:

By enhancing flexibility and strengthening the muscles surrounding the damaged joints, regular physical exercise helps treat chronic pain diseases like arthritis. Exercise also causes the production of endorphins, which have anti-anxiety and mood-lifting properties.

5. Improvement in Mental Health:

It has been shown that exercise improves cognitive function and lowers the chance of cognitive decline in older persons. It may raise brain health by enhancing memory, concentration, and processing speed. Additionally, exercise improves mental health by lowering stress, anxiety, and depressive symptoms.

6. Improved Sleeping Conditions:

Regular exercise may lengthen and improve the quality of sleep. Exercise helps older persons sleep longer and more deeply, which is crucial for maintaining their general health and vitality.

7. Social Participation:

Social connections are fostered by taking part in group fitness classes or other physical activities in the neighborhood. Feelings of loneliness and isolation, which are prevalent worries among older persons, may be combated by social connections, which are essential for mental well-being.

8. Improved Immune Function:

The immune system is strengthened by regular exercise, making the body more resistant to illnesses and infections. For older persons, whose immune systems may deteriorate with aging, this is particularly crucial.

Common Health Concerns in Seniors

1. Arthritis: Seniors often suffer from arthritis, a disorder that causes joint pain, stiffness, and swelling. The two most common kinds of arthritis, osteoarthritis and rheumatoid arthritis, both damage the joints and may impair movement.

2. Osteoporosis: Weak and brittle bones, which make them more prone to fractures and breaks, are symptoms of osteoporosis. If not treated appropriately, this illness, which is more common in older women, may cause serious health problems.

3. Heart disease: Seniors are more likely to develop heart disease, including coronary artery disease, atherosclerosis (hardening of the arteries), and hypertension (high blood pressure). Heart attacks and other cardiovascular issues may result from heart disease.

4. Diabetes: Diabetes type 2 is prevalent among elderly people. When the body stops producing enough insulin or develops resistance to it, high blood sugar levels result. Complications must be managed properly with food, exercise, and medicines.

5. Cancer: As people age, their chance of getting cancer rises. Lung, breast, colorectal, and prostate cancers are the most prevalent cancers among seniors. Cancer still poses a serious health risk, notwithstanding improvements brought about by early identification and medical advancements.

6. Alzheimer's disease and dementia: Seniors have a lot to worry about when it comes to cognitive decline, including Alzheimer's disease and other types of dementia. These illnesses have a profound influence on a person's quality of life and need considerable attention since they have an impact on memory, thinking, and conduct.

7. Depressive disorders and anxiety: Seniors often have mental health problems, such as sadness and anxiety, which are frequently made worse by things like loneliness, the death of a loved one, or long-term medical illnesses. These illnesses have a substantial impact on older individuals' general well-being and ability to go about their everyday lives.

8. Weight problems:

Obesity is a problem for seniors since it may cause a number of health difficulties, including diabetes, heart disease, and joint problems. It's essential to maintain a healthy weight through food and exercise to avoid the consequences of obesity.

9. Visual and auditory impairments:

Seniors often have eyesight and hearing loss due to aging. Diseases including macular degeneration, glaucoma, cataracts, and hearing loss might interfere with everyday living and activities.

10. Chronic Respiratory Conditions: As we age, breathing problems and decreased lung function are increasingly prevalent due to chronic obstructive pulmonary disease (COPD) and other respiratory disorders.

CHAPTER TWO

PREPARING FOR LOW IMPACT EXERCISES

Consultation with a Healthcare Professional

Our bodies change as we age, and as a result, so do our healthcare requirements. For preserving optimum health and addressing any potential issues, regular appointments with a healthcare practitioner, such as a primary care physician, geriatrician, or specialist, are essential. Seniors must schedule regular checkups and consultations for the following reasons:

1. Comprehensive Health Evaluation:

To understand your entire health, healthcare experts undertake extensive evaluations. They assess your medical history, do physical exams, and could order the required screenings and testing. This thorough assessment aids in identifying current health problems and determining your vulnerability to a range of illnesses.

2. Individualized health advice:

Healthcare specialists may provide specialized guidance tailored to your unique requirements based on their evaluation of your health. This could include suggestions for dietary changes, physical activity, medication management, and preventative actions. With individualized support, you can be confident that your healthcare strategy fits your particular needs.

3. Manage chronic conditions:

Many elderly people deal with long-term medical concerns, including diabetes, hypertension, or arthritis. Healthcare experts ensure that drugs are changed as necessary and lifestyle adjustments are made to enhance your quality of life in order to properly manage chronic disorders.

4. Early Detection of Health Issues:

Routine checkups allow for the early identification of possible health issues. Early problem detection often enables simpler, more efficient treatments, reducing problems and increasing results.

5. Vaccinations and Preventive Care:

Professionals in the medical field provide crucial preventative treatments, such as immunizations against the flu, pneumonia, and other illnesses. Seniors in particular need to have these immunizations because they improve the immune system's capacity to combat infections and lower the risk of serious diseases.

6. Medication Administration:

Seniors often take a number of drugs. Medical specialists check your drugs to make sure they're effective and safe, avoiding any combinations or side effects. Additionally, they may alter prescriptions or modify doses as needed.

7. Support for emotional and mental health:

Healthcare experts can evaluate your emotional and mental health. If necessary, they may provide advice, support, and referrals to mental health professionals. As crucial as controlling physical health, addressing mental health issues

8. Coordination of Care:

Your treatment is coordinated by medical personnel, particularly if you see many specialists. They provide a holistic approach to your well-being by making sure that all facets of your health are taken into account.

Choosing the Right Exercise Gear

For seniors in particular, choosing the right equipment is essential to comfort, safety, and efficacy throughout your workout regimen.

Seniors' Guide to Choosing the Right Exercise Equipment

1. Wearing comfortable shoes is important:

Spend money on supportive, well-fitting sporting shoes with enough arch support and cushioning. To avoid foot discomfort, give stability, and lower the chance of falling during activities, it is important to choose comfortable shoes.

2. Clothes that are breathable and moisture-wicking:

Choose textiles that drain away perspiration from your body to keep you dry and comfortable. During exercises, loose-fitting, breathable clothing helps control body temperature while allowing for full range of motion.

3. Wear the proper socks:

Select cushioned, blister-free socks that wick away moisture. Proper socks and well-fitting shoes improve foot comfort, especially while moving about or doing aerobic workouts.

4. Supportive Bras:

Invest in supportive sports bras that limit breast mobility and provide sufficient support for women during physical activity. In order to feel comfortable and avoid stress on the back and chest, the breasts must be supported properly.

5. Gloves and wrist support:

Consider using gloves to protect your hands and improve your grip while weightlifting or using resistance bands. Wrist support bands may also be helpful while doing activities that call for wrist stability.

6. Safety accessories include:

Consider safety equipment like knee or elbow pads depending on your training regimen, particularly if you do activities that require you to lie on your stomach or in a prone posture. These add-ons provide additional padding and safeguard joints.

7. Appropriate Eyewear:

If you use glasses, be sure you have impact-resistant lenses and safe frames for sports. Sunglasses with UV protection protect your eyes from dangerous sun rays while participating in outdoor activities.

8. Pedometer or fitness tracker:

You may track your steps, track your activity levels, and track your progress with the use of a fitness tracker or pedometer. Many contemporary fitness trackers are easy to use and may provide you with useful information about your exercises and general health.

9. Water Bottle:

By keeping a handy, spill-proof water bottle close at hand, you can stay hydrated while exercising. Maintaining energy levels and sustaining general physiological processes require proper hydration.

10. Consultation with a Specialist:

Consider speaking with a physical therapist or exercise professional if you have certain health issues or ailments. They may advise on customized equipment or adjustments made just for you, guaranteeing a secure and efficient training program.

Creating a Safe Exercise Space at Home

It's crucial to set up a secure workout area at home, particularly for seniors who wish to participate in regular physical activity.

1. Purge the area: Start by removing any debris, furniture, and other obstructions from the specified workout area. Ensure there is sufficient space to move about without running the danger of stumbling or bumping against things.

2. Select an Area with Good Lighting: Exercise in a well-lit area for improved vision and a lower accident risk. While exercising inside is preferable, utilize bright, energy-efficient LED or daylight-toned lamps to light the space.

3. Utilize non-slip flooring: Choose non-slip flooring materials such as rubber mats, yoga mats, or interlocking foam tiles. These materials provide traction, making it safer to exercise without the worry of sliding, particularly while engaging in balance-related activities.

4. Secure Carpets & Rugs: If there are carpets or rugs in the workout area, ensure they are fastened with double-sided tape or non-slip pads. Rugs that are too loose or wrinkled might be dangerous and lead to slips and falls.

5. Strong furnishings and supporting tools:

Make sure the furniture or workout equipment you use is solid and steady. Purchase sturdy furniture that can hold your weight and actions without toppling over, such as chairs, tables, or workout equipment.

6. Accessible emergency supplies: A first-aid kit, a phone, and emergency contacts should all be kept close at hand. Having rapid access to these goods is essential in the event of any accidents or medical crises.

7. Appropriate Ventilation: Maintain a healthy airflow in the workout area. Proper ventilation, particularly while engaging in strenuous activity, aids in temperature regulation and avoids overheating. For better air circulation, think about turning on fans or opening windows.

8. Having sufficient heating and cooling: Make sure the temperature is appropriate for the space. You will be encouraged to exercise consistently without suffering if your home is properly heated in the winter and cooled in the summer.

9. Mirror for Form Check: Put a mirror in the workout area if you can. When exercising, you may use a mirror to examine your form and posture, which can help you maintain appropriate technique and avoid injuries.

10. Storage for Equipment: Cleanly arrange your exercise equipment. When not in use, keep weights, resistance bands, and other equipment organized and out of the way by using shelves, baskets, or storage bins.

11. Regular Safety Checks: Check the workout area often for damage. Mats that are damaged should be changed, furniture should be stable, and lights should be working properly. A secure workout environment is maintained by regular safety assessments.

CHAPTER THREE

WARM-UP AND COOL-DOWN ROUTINES

Importance of Warm-Up Exercises

Regardless of age or fitness level, warm-up activities are an essential part of any workout regimen. These easy exercises, done at the start of a workout, are crucial in getting the body ready for harder physical activity.

1. Increased blood flow:

Exercises for warming up help circulate more blood and raise the heart rate gradually. Your muscles get more oxygen and nutrients from this increased blood flow, which helps them get ready for the forthcoming activity. The danger of cardiovascular stress during the primary workout session is also decreased because of improved blood circulation.

2. Improved Muscle Flexibility:

Stretching is a component of warm-up activities that helps increase joint and muscle range of motion. Exercises requiring correct form and technique are simpler to do when muscles and joints are flexible and less prone to injury.

3. Reduced Muscle Stiffness:

Your muscles tend to stiffen as you age, making them more susceptible to sprains and injuries. Warm-up exercises aid in easing these tight muscles, enhancing their flexibility and responsiveness to motion.

4. Injury Prevention:

The prevention of injuries is one of the main goals of warm-up activities. Warm-ups enable your muscles, tendons, and ligaments to progressively adapt to the motions by preparing your body for the approaching physical activity. Strains, sprains, and other injuries are less likely as a result of this training.

5. Improved Joint Lubrication:

Exercises that warm you up increase the flow of synovial fluid into your joints. This liquid functions as a lubricant, lowering friction and enabling pain-free fluid motions between the joints. For older people to preserve joint health, proper joint lubrication is particularly crucial.

6. The sixth point is mental readiness:

A brief period of concentrated, conscious movement is offered by warm-up activities. You may mentally get ready for the workout at this time, which will improve your focus and motivation throughout the actual exercise session.

7. Better Balance and Coordination:

Balance and coordination drills are often included in warming-up exercises. As your proprioception (awareness of your body's location in space) improves, you'll have better balance and a lower chance of falling, which is a major issue for seniors.

8. Gradual Elevation of Heart Rate:

Warm-ups assist in gradually raising your heart rate. Without a thorough warm-up, sudden, intensive physical exercise may strain your heart and possibly cause cardiovascular issues, particularly in older people.

9. Faster Muscle Relaxation and Contraction:

Exercises that warm up your muscles help them contract and release more quickly. Your performance throughout the primary exercise will be increased, and the chance of muscular cramps will be decreased thanks to this greater muscle reactivity.

Low Impact Stretching and Flexibility Exercises

Any fitness regimen must include stretching and flexibility exercises, particularly for older citizens. These low-impact exercises help with flexibility as well as joint mobility, muscle stiffness reduction, and general wellbeing. Here is a guide to adding low-impact flexibility and stretching activities to your daily schedule:

1. Stretches for the neck: Rotate your neck in a circle and gently tilt your head from side to side, forward and back. These exercises improve neck flexibility and decrease stiffness while releasing tension in the shoulders and neck.

2. Shoulders roll: Roll your shoulders in a circle, forward and back. This exercise facilitates neck and upper back muscular relaxation while enhancing shoulder mobility and reducing stiffness.

3. Stretching the wrist and arms: Flex and stretch your wrists lightly as you raise your arms in front of you. Holding each stretch for a little while. Those who spend a lot of time typing or writing can benefit from these exercises since they increase wrist and forearm flexibility.

4. Chest Opening Stretch: Straighten your arms, stand tall, and clasp your hands behind your back. Open your chest by lifting your arms just a little. For 15 to 30 seconds, maintain the stretch. This stretch encourages chest and shoulder flexibility while correcting forward-slumping posture.

5. Spinal twists: Place your feet flat on the floor while sitting on a chair. While supporting yourself with the chair's backrest, gradually twist your body to one side. After holding for a few breaths, switch to the other side. Spinal twists increase the spine's range of motion and improve posture.

6: Sitting leg raises Sit in a chair with your feet flat on the floor and your back straight. One leg should be raised straight in front of you, held for a brief period of time, and then brought back down. the other leg, and repeat. This workout strengthens the quadriceps while increasing hamstring flexibility.

7. Stretching the calf:

Approximately an arm's length away, face the wall. Put your right foot straight behind you and plant your heel into the ground. Switch to the other leg after holding the stretch for 15 to 30 seconds. Calf exercises improve lower leg flexibility and help keep muscles from becoming stiff.

8. Squatting Butterfly Stretch: With your feet together and your back straight, take a seat on the ground. Hold your feet while bending your knees slightly toward the floor. This stretch increases hip flexibility and is very helpful for elderly people who have hip joint problems.

9. Ankle Roll: Lift one foot off the ground while you comfortably sit or stand. Rotate your ankle in a clockwise and counterclockwise direction. With this workout, your ankles will move more freely and feel less stiff.

10. Deep breathing and stretching:

Include deep breathing when stretching. As you prepare to stretch your muscles, take a deep breath and let it out as you do so. Your stretches will be more effective since deep breathing helps to relax the body.

Cooling Down Safely: Post-Exercise Stretches

Warming up before physical exercise and cooling down are both crucial. Stretching after exercise aids your body's transition from an active to a resting state, encouraging muscular relaxation and flexibility. Here is a list of secure and efficient stretching exercises for seniors after exercise:

1. Hamstring Extensor Stretch:

The sole of your foot should contact the inside of your thigh while you sit on the floor with one leg straight and the other leg bent. Maintaining a straight back, bend forward toward your toes. For 20 to 30 seconds, hold. On the other side, repeat. Flexibility in the hamstrings is improved by this stretch.

2. Stretching the quadriceps:

Hold onto a chair or a wall for support while you stand erect. Bring your heel near your buttocks while bending one knee. Hold your ankle in place for 20 to 30 seconds with a soft grip. Change to the other leg. The quadriceps muscles on the front of your thighs are the focus of this stretch.

3. Stretching the calf:

Put your hands against the wall as you stand facing it. Step back with one foot, keeping it straight, and plant your heel firmly on the ground. For 20 to 30 seconds, maintain the stretch on the other leg, and repeat. To avoid stiffness and cramping in the lower leg muscles, calf stretches are crucial.

4 Stretching the hip flexors:

Make a 90-degree angle by kneeling on one knee with the other foot in front. Keep your back straight and gently move your hips forward. For 20 to 30 seconds, maintain the stretch. Change to the other side. The muscles at the front of your hips and thighs are the focus of this stretch.

5. Squatting Forward Bend:

Legs straight in front of you, sit down on the floor. Maintaining a flat back, extend your front arm toward your toes. For 20 to 30 seconds, maintain the stretch. The hamstrings and lower back become more flexible with this stretch.

6. Children's Pose:

Start on your knees, raise your heels, and sit back while keeping your arms out in front of you. Hold the stretch while concentrating on taking deep breaths and unwinding into the position. The lower back and hips may be stretched well in a child's pose.

7. Stretching the triceps:

Reach your hand down your back with one arm raised above, elbow bent. Gently squeeze your bent elbow with your other hand. For 20 to 30 seconds, hold. Change to the other arm. The triceps muscles at the rear of your upper arms are the focus of this stretch.

8. Stretching the neck and shoulders:

Bring your ear nearer your shoulder as you gently incline your head to one side. For 15 to 20 seconds, hold. On the other side, repeat. Bring one arm across your body and use the hand on the other side to slowly draw it toward your chest to extend your shoulders. For 20 to 30 seconds, hold. Change to the other arm.

9. Deep Breathing and Relaxation:

Spend a few minutes in deep breathing and relaxation to round off your stretching regimen after your workout. Close your eyes, choose a comfortable seat or lay down, and concentrate on your breathing. Take a big breath in with your nose, hold it for a second, and then gently let it out through your mouth. Following an exercise, this relaxation method aids in body and mental relaxation.

10. Hydrogenate and replenish:

Make sure to replenish your body by consuming water or another hydrating beverage after your stretches. To help with muscle rehabilitation, think about consuming a small snack that is high in protein and carbs.

CHAPTER FOUR

CARDIOVASCULAR EXERCISES

Gentle Aerobic Activities for Seniors

Regular aerobic exercise is essential for preserving cardiovascular health, stamina, and general wellbeing, particularly in older people. Here is a list of mild cardio exercises suitable for senior citizens:

1. Walking:

Low-impact aerobic exercise like walking is simple to include in your regular schedule. On most days of the week, try to walk briskly for at least 30 minutes. To make your walks pleasurable, use attractive pathways or routes in parks.

2. Swimming:

Excellent low-impact workouts that are gentle on the joints include swimming and water aerobics. Multiple muscle groups are worked by swimming, which also increases flexibility and cardiovascular fitness. Participate in a water aerobics class at your neighborhood pool.

3. cycling:

Seniors might choose stationary bikes or flat-terrain riding outside. Cycling offers good cardiovascular exercise while being easy on the joints. Start with a low-resistance setting on a stationary bike and progressively raise the intensity as your stamina improves.

4. Dancing:

In addition to improving your cardio fitness, dancing also makes your training more enjoyable. Attend senior-focused dancing lessons, or just turn on your favorite music and dance around your living room. It's a fantastic approach to raising your cardiovascular health, balance, and coordination.

5. Exercises for the chair:

Sitting for aerobic activities may be quite beneficial for seniors who have trouble moving about or maintaining their balance. Excellent alternatives include sat-tap dancing, seated leg lifts, and seated marches. These activities support maintaining muscular tone and good heart health.

6. Tai Chi:

Deep breathing and slow, flowing motions merge in Tai Chi, a peaceful and elegant type of exercise. It encourages relaxation and stress reduction while enhancing balance, flexibility, and strength. There are several senior-focused Tai Chi courses offered.

7. Low-Impact Aerobic Classes:

Low-impact aerobics courses designed for elders are widely available in fitness facilities and community organizations. These courses often include stretching, weight training, and aerobic activities. For lessons near you, check the classifieds in your region.

8. Gardening:

Despite popular belief, gardening may be a great aerobic exercise. Your heart rate may be raised, and a low-impact exercise is provided by digging, planting, and even light yard labor. Just be aware of how your body moves and try not to push yourself too much.

9. Mini Trampoline with Rebounder:

Rebounding on a small trampoline, or rebounder, offers a low-impact cardio exercise. Balance, coordination, and cardiovascular fitness are all enhanced by light trampoline bouncing. Use the trampoline on a level, non-slip surface, and make sure it is stable.

10. Golf:

Walking the course while playing golf provides some modest cardio exercise. Even though it may not be very demanding, strolling from hole to hole offers a regular, low-impact workout. Just keep in mind to carry your stuff or, for additional convenience, utilize a pull cart.

Walking and Nordic Walking Techniques

Walking, one of the most basic but efficient kinds of exercise, has several positive health effects. Walking poles are used in Nordic walking, a variant of regular walking that works the upper body muscles.

1. Walking:

Standing tall with your head up and shoulders back is the proper posture. To lessen strain on your back, keep your spine neutral and straight.

As you walk, let your arms hang loose and swing as they naturally do.

To stabilize your posture, contract your core muscles.

Foot Position:

- With each stride, begin on your heel and roll through the ball of your foot to your toes.

- Move naturally, not too quickly or slowly. Your step should be relaxed and effective.
- Try not to drag your steps to lessen the chance of stumbling.

Breathing:

- Take many slow, rhythmic breaths. Use your nose to take in air and your mouth to let it out.
- Pay attention to your breathing to make sure you're receiving enough oxygen, particularly while you're vigorously walking.

2. Nordic Walking Methodology

The use of walking poles when Nordic walking activates the muscles in the upper body and works the whole body.

Holding the Poles:

- Grip the poles firmly yet comfortably. Your elbows need to be just slightly bent to allow for easy movement. Your hands should just loosely grasp the handles since the poles should be inclined rearward.
- Plant the poles behind you as you go ahead (pole placement). With each step, press down on the poles to advance yourself.

- Sync up your leg and arm motions. Your left pole should be grounded while your right foot advances, and the opposite is true.

Engaging Upper Body Muscles:

- As you press down on the poles, use your shoulders, arms, and back muscles.

- Concentrate on creating a flowing motion by engaging your full body. Your arms should resemble an extension of the poles.

- Starting at a comfortable rate, gradually increase your speed as your fitness level rises. This is the recommended walking speed and intensity.

- Nordic walking may be adjusted for various degrees of effort. Increase your walking pace or include steep terrain for a harder exercise.

Safety Advice:

- Be aware of your surroundings, particularly if you're going through busy places or on uneven ground.

- To avoid sliding, use suitable footwear with strong traction.

- If you're new to exercising, start with shorter sessions and gradually increase the length and intensity to prevent overexertion.

Seated Cardio Workouts for Limited Mobility

Exercise for the heart doesn't have to be abandoned because of limited mobility. For those with mobility issues, seated cardio exercises are a great method to preserve cardiovascular health, increase circulation, and enhance general wellbeing.

1. Sitting and marching:

Straighten your back while sitting on the edge of a firm chair. Alternating between bringing one knee up to your chest and bringing it back down Up the tempo for an additional aerobic challenge. To improve stability when marching, contract your core muscles.

2. Squatting Leg Extensions:

Straighten your feet and adopt a tall posture. Straighten one leg out in front of you, keep it there for a while, then lower it. Legs should be switched while maintaining controlled motions. Use ankle weights to increase the intensity.

3. Seated tap dancing:

As you tap your feet on the floor in alternating directions, choose a comfortable seat. Tap your heels, toes, or both. Make it fun by listening to upbeat music, and quicken the pace to help your heart.

4. Sitting and Jumping Jacks:

Your arms should be at your sides when you sit with your back straight. Jump your arms aloft and spread your legs wide before returning to the starting position. To raise your heart rate, do this exercise while sitting.

5. Sitting Side Taps:

Put your feet flat on the floor and sit down. Alternate between tapping your left hand to your right hip and your right hand to your left hip. For a sitting aerobic exercise, use your oblique muscles and raise the pace.

6. Seat-based cycling:

Utilize a seated elliptical machine or stationary pedal exerciser. Comfortably position yourself in a pedaling position. The cardiovascular system and leg strength both greatly benefit from this low-impact exercise.

7. Sitting and Rowing:

Straighten your feet and adopt a tall posture. With both hands, hold a resistance or workout band in front of you.

Use your back muscles to pull the band closer to your chest. Repeat after a slow release. The upper body gets a tremendous cardiac workout from this sitting rowing action.

8. Seated boxing:

Hold a few light weights in your hands, or none at all. Punching forward and switching arms while seated are boxing motions. For a successful cardio exercise, keep your motions regulated and rhythmic while engaging your core.

9. Sitting Down and Dancing:

Play your preferred music and jive while seated! As the music beats, move your hips, torso, and arms accordingly. Not only can dancing improve your cardiovascular health, but it also makes exercise more fun and uplifts your mood.

10. Deep Breathing Exercises:

Deep breathing exercises enhance lung capacity while increasing oxygen intake, even though they are not conventional cardio activities. Inhale deeply through your nose, then slowly exhale through your mouth while sitting comfortably. Increase the length of your breaths progressively while concentrating on getting air into your lungs.

CHAPTER FIVE

STRENGTH AND BALANCE EXERCISES

Chair-Based Strength Training Exercises

Seniors must engage in strength exercise because it maintains muscle mass, increases bone density, and improves mobility. Chair-based strength training may be a safe and efficient technique to increase strength and endurance if you have restricted mobility or prefer sitting activities. Here is a list of senior-specific chair-based strength training exercises:

1. Squatting leg lifts:

Place your feet flat on the ground and sit on the edge of a solid chair. One leg should be raised straight out in front of you, held for a while, then brought back down. Continue with the opposite leg. To build up your quadriceps, do 10-15 reps on each leg.

2. Sitting Marching:

Sit upright and raise your knees as high as is comfortable while keeping your legs in place. Keep a quick pace and use your core muscles. March for one to two minutes to strengthen your legs and cardiovascular system.

3. Squats with heel raises:

Straighten your feet and adopt a tall posture. While keeping your toes on the ground, lift your heels. After a little pause, bring your heels back down. Use 15-20 reps to work the calf muscles.

4. Sitting Knee Extensions:

Your feet should be level on the floor, and your back should be straight. Lift your foot a few inches off the ground while extending one knee. After a little pause, drop your foot back down. Continue with the opposite leg. To strengthen your hamstrings, try to complete 10 to 15 repetitions on each leg.

5. Squatting Leg Press:

Place your back against the chair's backrest when you sit down. your thighs with your hands there. Using your leg muscles, push your hands and thighs together. Hold for a little while, then let go. Work your inner thighs and quadriceps by doing 10–15 repetitions.

6. Squatting Chest Press:

With both hands, hold a tiny ball or a pillow at chest height. Put your hands together and tense your chest. Hold for a little while before letting go. To make your chest muscles stronger, do 10-15 repetitions.

7. Squatting Shoulder Press:

With your elbows bent, hold a small weight (or water bottles) in each hand at shoulder height. Up until your arms are completely extended, lift the weights. Return the weights to shoulder height. Work your shoulder muscles by doing 10–15 repetitions.

8. Seated Bicep Curls:

Your arms should be stretched downward while you hold a weight in each hand. As you pull the weights closer to your shoulders, bend your elbows. Reverse the weights' descent. Target your bicep muscles by doing 10–15 reps.

9. Sitting Triceps Dips

Your hands should be on the front edge of the chair, pointing down toward your feet. Bending your elbows allows you to lower your torso a few inches while lifting your hips off the chair. Return to the starting position by pushing up. To build up your tricep muscles, do 10-15 repetitions.

10. Squatting abdominal twists while seated:

Straighten your feet and adopt a tall posture. With both hands, hold a pillow or ball at chest height. Engage your oblique muscles as you turn your torso first to the right, then to the left. To strengthen your abdominal muscles, practice 15-20 twists on each side.

Resistance Band Workouts

Exercises using resistance bands provide a practical and customizable technique to improve your general fitness and strength. Resistance bands offer moderate but effective resistance, making them a good choice for muscle development, enhancing mobility, and boosting joint stability. They are suitable for people of all fitness levels, including seniors. You may add the following resistance band workouts to your fitness regimen:

1. Banded Squats:

Just above your knees, wrap the resistance band across your thighs. Place your feet shoulder-width apart as you stand. Squat down while maintaining a straight back and an uplifted chest. In order to go back to the beginning position, drive through your heels. Your glutes, hamstrings, and quads will all benefit from this workout.

2. Banded Rows:

Stretch your legs out straight in front of you as you sit down on the floor. Holding the ends with both hands, wrap the resistance band around the bottoms of your feet. Pull the band towards your waist while keeping your back straight and pulling your shoulder blades together. Repeat after letting go. Your shoulders and back will be strengthened by this workout.

3. Banded Chest Press:

The resistance band should be fastened around a strong post at chest level. Keeping your hands apart and away from the anchor point, hold the band handles. Step forward to increase the band's tension. Until your arms are completely extended, move both of your arms forward. Return to the starting position gradually. Your chest muscles are the focus of this workout.

4. Banded Leg Raises:

The resistance band should be wrapped around your ankles while you lay on your back. Lift your legs up toward the ceiling while keeping them straight, then bring them down a few inches off the ground. During the whole exercise, contract your core muscles. The lower abdominal muscles are worked during this workout.

5. Blocked Shoulder Press:

Place your feet shoulder-width apart and stand in the middle of the resistance band. Hold the band handles with your hands facing forward and at shoulder height. Press the bands while raising your arms completely. Back down to shoulder height with the bands. Your shoulder muscles become stronger with this workout.

6. Banded lateral raises:

Place your feet hip-width apart and stand in the middle of the resistance band. With your hands toward your thighs, hold the band handles by your sides. Reach shoulder height by raising your arms out to the sides. Your arms should now be at your sides. Your lateral deltoids are the focus of this workout.

7. Banded Leg Press:

Stretch your legs out straight in front of you as you sit down on the floor. Holding the band handles in your hands, loop the resistance band around your feet. Extend your legs straight out after bending your knees and bringing them up to your chest. Repeat this motion while using your abdominal muscles. Your quadriceps and lower abdominal muscles are worked throughout this workout.

8. Bicep curls using bands:

Stand with your feet shoulder-width apart on the resistance band. Your arms should be completely extended while you hold the band handles with your palms facing forward. Curl the bands toward your shoulders while keeping your upper arms still to squeeze your biceps. Return the bands to the starting position gradually.

9. Banded tricep extensions:

Raise your right arm above while holding the resistance band's one end in your right hand. Bring your hand behind your head while bending your elbow. Reach behind your back with your left hand and grasp the opposite end of the band. Your right arm should be straight and pointed upward. Returning to the initial posture, bend your arm. Next, switch hands again.

10. Banded Woodchoppers:

The doorknob, for example, is a good place to anchor the resistance band. Standing with your feet shoulder-width apart, face the anchor point. With both hands at your hips, hold the band handle. Raise your arms diagonally across your body, terminating over the shoulder on the other side, while rotating your torso while maintaining straight arms. Repeat from your starting position.

Balance Exercises to Prevent Falls

For seniors in particular, maintaining excellent balance is essential since it lowers the chance of falling and improves mobility in general. Your stability and confidence may dramatically increase by adding balancing exercises to your program. To help avoid falls, try these efficient balancing exercises:

1. Single-Legged Stands

Hold onto anything for support while you stand behind a strong chair or a tabletop. Lift your left foot a few inches off the ground as you shift your weight to your right leg. For 10 to 15 seconds, maintain this posture, then move to the other leg. Try to extend each balancing hold's time as you go.

2. Walking from heel to toe:

Consider yourself on a tightrope. Your left foot's toes should be behind the heel of your right foot. As you walk in a straight path, concentrate on a point in front of you to maintain equilibrium. Take 20 steps, then go the other way and come back. You may use a wall or a countertop as support if necessary.

3. Exercises for Balance on One Leg:

For support, cling to a firm surface. Aim for 10 to 30 seconds while raising one leg off the ground and maintaining the posture. As your stability increases, test yourself by balancing on one leg while shutting your eyes as you go.

4. Marching in Place:

Place your feet hip-width apart and stand tall. Swing your arms softly and raise your knees high, as if you were marching. Maintain a straight spine and contract your core muscles. To increase balance and coordination, march in place for a few seconds.

5. Walking a tightrope:

A straight line on the floor comes to mind. Put one foot in front of the other as you go down this line. Keep your eyes on a distant object and keep your balance while you move. Your steadiness will be tested throughout this workout, which also tones your legs.

6. Weight Changes:

Place your feet hip-width apart as you stand. Lift your left foot off the ground while you gradually transfer your weight to your right foot. Hold for a brief moment, then lift your right foot and shift your weight to your left foot. Continue shifting your weight while maintaining controlled and fluid motions. Put in 10 to 15 shifts per leg.

7. Clock Reach:

Think of yourself as being in the middle of a clock. Lift one leg and point your arms in the direction of various clock times (for instance, 12, 3, and 9 o'clock). Hold each posture for a short while, then go to the other leg. Your ability to reach in diverse directions is improved, and your balance is improved with this exercise.

8. Using the stork's stands:

Lift the opposite foot while standing on one leg, bending your knee, and bringing the foot closer to your buttocks. For 10 to 15 seconds, maintain this one-legged balance. Repeat on the other leg after switching. Consider shutting your eyes while balancing for extra difficulty.

9. Exercises on a balance board or wobble board:

To put your stability to the test even further, use a balancing board or wobble board. As the board tilts, attempt to stand on it while keeping your balance. Start with little tilts and build up your range of motion as your confidence grows.

10. Tai Chi and Yoga:

Consider engaging in yoga or Tai Chi, which both place an emphasis on flexibility, balance, and mindful movement. By enhancing your balance, coordination, and general body awareness, these age-old techniques help lower your chance of falling.

CHAPTER SIX

FLEXIBILITY AND MOBILITY EXERCISES

Gentle Yoga and Tai Chi for Seniors

Both Tai Chi and gentle yoga are age-old arts that improve the body and mind in a variety of ways, making them excellent for older citizens. These exercises encourage flexibility, balance, and general well-being by emphasizing slow, gentle movements, breathing exercises, and awareness.

Gentle Yoga for Seniors

1. Chair Yoga:

Traditional yoga postures are modified in chair yoga so that they may be performed while seated or with the assistance of a chair. This exercise promotes circulation, muscular strength, and flexibility. Poses for chair yoga might include breathing exercises, moderate stretches, and sitting twists.

2. Standing yoga positions:

Standing yoga postures help enhance balance and stability in seniors who can support themselves while standing. With the use of a chair or wall for balance support, poses like Mountain Pose (Tadasana), Tree

Pose (Vrksasana), and Warrior Pose (Virabhadrasana) may be modified.

3. Gently stretch your muscles.

Concentrate on light stretching motions that target large muscle groups. Stretching increases flexibility, eases joint pain, and reduces muscular stiffness. Include sitting forward bends, shoulder rolls, and neck stretches in your program.

4. Exercises for Breathing (Pranayama):

Deep breathing techniques should be used to expand lung capacity and encourage calm. Stress may be reduced and the mind can be calmed using breathing methods like alternate nostril breathing and diaphragmatic breathing.

5. Mental health and mindfulness:

Give yourself some time to practice mindfulness and meditation. Stress reduction and improved mental clarity may result from guided meditation sessions that emphasize relaxation and positive affirmations.

Seniors and Tai Chi

1. Exercises to Warm Up With:

Start your Tai Chi practice with some easy stretching. Hip rotations, shoulder circles, and neck rotations are a few examples. Exercises that warm up the body get it ready for Tai Chi's fluid motions.

2. Tai Chi forms include:

Learn and practice the Tai Chi forms that have been simplified for elders. These forms include slow, fluid motions that enhance flexibility, balance, and coordination. The motions encourage harmony and are often inspired by nature.

3. Exercises for weight shifting and balance:

Weight shifting and deliberate motions, which are emphasized in tai chi, improve stability and balance. Practice shifting your weight from one leg to the other while progressively extending your range of motion. Leg stability and strength are encouraged by balance exercises like "Golden Rooster Stands on One Leg".

4. Breathing and relaxation:

During Tai Chi practice, pay attention to deep, diaphragmatic breathing. Moving in sync with your breath improves attention and relaxation. Tai Chi integrates the idea of "qi," or energy flow, directing the breath to encourage a feeling of serenity and concentration.

5. Relaxing and practicing meditation:

Finish your Tai Chi practice with some easy stretching and seated meditation. Think about your physical feelings and the serenity of the exercise. Tai chi meditation improves inner calm and self-awareness.

Stretching Exercises for Improved Flexibility

Every workout regimen should include stretching since it helps with flexibility, range of motion, and injury prevention. You can maintain and enhance your flexibility by including a range of stretching activities in your regular regimen. Here is a list of stretches that emphasize general flexibility while concentrating on certain muscle groups:

1. **Neck stretch:**

- Stretch your neck by standing or sitting tall and keeping your shoulders relaxed.
- To feel a light stretch on the other side of your neck, tilt your head to one side and push your ear up toward your shoulder.
- Hold for 15 to 30 seconds before alternating to the opposite side.

- You may gently lay your palm on your head and apply mild pressure to lengthen the stretch.

2. Shoulder Extensor Stretch:

- Cross your right arm firmly over your chest.
- Holding your right arm at the elbow with your left hand, slowly bring it toward your chest.
- Feel the stretch in your shoulder and the back of your arm as you hold for 15 to 30 seconds.
- Continue on the other side.

3. Triceps Stretch:

- To stretch your triceps, raise your right arm above, bend your elbow, and extend your hand behind your back.
- Gently prod your right elbow with your left hand.
- Maintain the stretch along your triceps and the back of your arm for 15 to 30 seconds.
- Repeat with the other arm.

4. Chest Opening Stretch:

- Place your feet hip-width apart and stand tall.
- Straighten your arms and clasp your hands behind your back.
- Squeeze your shoulder blades together, lift your arms a little, and open your chest.

- Maintain the stretch over your shoulders and chest for 15 to 30 seconds.

5. Stretch your wrists and forearms:

- Straighten your right arm in front of you, palm down.

- Gently push down with your left hand on your fingers to extend your wrist and forearm.

- Continue holding for 15–30 seconds before switching to the other hand.

- Extend your arm with the palm facing up, and repeat the stretch on the opposite side.

6. Sitting Forward Bend:

- Sit on the ground with your legs straight out in front of you.

- Take a deep breath in, stretch your spine, and let it out as you hinge at the hips and reach your toes.

- According to your flexibility, hold onto your shins, ankles, or feet.

- Feel the stretch in your hamstrings and lower back as you hold the stretch for 30 to 1 minute.

7. Quadriceps Stretch:

- Holding your right heel with your right hand, stand tall and move it toward your buttocks.
- Maintain a tight knee range of motion and straight thighs.
- Hold for 15 to 30 seconds while allowing the front of your thigh to extend.
- Continue on the other side.

8. Squatting Butterfly Stretch:

- Kneel down with your feet together and your knees slightly bent.
- Holding your feet in place with your hands, slowly lower your knees to the floor.
- Sit up straight and feel the stretch in your inner thighs and hips for 30 seconds.

9. Calf Stretch:

- Place your hands against the wall while you stand facing it.
- Step back with your right foot, keeping it straight, and plant your heel firmly on the ground.
- Feel the stretch in your calf muscles and hold the stretch for 15 to 30 seconds.
- Repeat with the other leg.

10. Stretching the quadratus lumborum while standing:

- Cross your right ankle over your left while you stand with your feet hip-width apart.
- Raise your right arm above while bending your left torso.
- Feel the stretch down the side of your body and hold the stretch for 15 to 30 seconds.
- Move to the other side, then repeat.

Tips for Safe Stretching:

- Warm up your body with a brief bout of aerobic exercise before stretching to improve blood flow to your muscles.
- Stretch softly and slowly; do not bounce or make sudden motions.
- To help your muscles relax, breathe deeply and steadily during each stretch.
- Pay attention to the muscles you're stretching, and pay attention to any tightness or pain you may feel.
- Avoid overextending your stretches; they should be pleasant and just slightly difficult.

- To encourage the muscles to loosen up and lengthen, hold each stretch for at least 15 to 30 seconds.

Enhancing Mobility with Range of Motion Exercises

Range-of-motion exercises are intended to lengthen your muscles and loosen your joints, improving your general mobility and lowering your risk of accidents. For older people, those who are healing from injuries, or anybody who wants to increase their flexibility, these exercises are particularly crucial. Here is a list of range-of-motion exercises for different body parts:

1. Rotations of the neck

- Keep your back straight while you stand or sit.
- Turn your head slowly to the right as far as it will go, then bring it back to the middle.
- Continue on the left side.
- To improve neck mobility, do 10–15 repetitions on each side.

2. Shoulders roll:

- Place your feet shoulder-width apart when standing.

- Raise your shoulders up toward your ears, then gently roll them back.
- Turn the movement around and roll your shoulders forward.
- Roll your shoulders for 10–15 counts in each direction to increase range of motion.

3. Arm Circumferences:

- Arms outstretched to the sides.
- Begin by making little circles with your arms and enlarging them with time.
- After 10 to 15 revolutions, reverse the orientation of the circles.
- Arm circles promote blood flow to the arms and shoulder flexibility.

4. Stretching the wrist flexors and tendons:

- Straighten out your right arm and place your palm downward.
- Gently push down with your left hand on your fingers to extend your wrist and forearm.
- Hold for 15 to 30 seconds before moving to the other hand.
- To target other muscles in your forearm, reverse the stretch while holding your palm upward.

5. Hip Circumference:

- Place your hands on your hips as you stand.

- Circularly rotate your hips, first clockwise and then counterclockwise.

- Make 10 to 15 circles in each direction, paying attention to your motions.

- Hip circles enhance hip flexibility and mobility.

6. Knee Flexion and Extension:

- Place your feet flat on the ground while seated on a chair.

- Lift your right foot slowly off the ground while attempting to keep your knee as straight as you can.

- After a little period of holding, bring your foot back down.

- Do the same with your left foot.

- Perform 10–15 reps on each leg to make your knees more flexible.

7. Ankle Alphabet:

- Lie down or sit with your legs fully extended.

- Raise your right foot just a little bit above the ground, then spin your ankle to form the alphabet's letters in the air.
- Do the same with your left foot.
- This exercise strengthens the muscles around the joint and increases ankle mobility.

8. Sitting leg raises:

- Straighten your back while seated on the edge of a chair.
- Straighten out your right leg, then raise it as high as is comfortable.
- After a little pause, bring your leg back down.
- the left leg, then repeat.
- To improve hip and thigh flexibility, elevate your legs 10–15 times each.

9. Spinal Twists:

- Place your feet flat on the floor or cross them in front of you while sitting in a chair.
- Put your left hand on the ground behind you and your right hand on your left knee.
- Tilt your body to the left and glance to your left.
- Hold for 15 to 30 seconds before alternating to the opposite side.

- Spinal twists promote thoracic rotation and increase the spine's flexibility.

10. Deep Breathing Exercises:

- Take a comfy seat or lay down.
- Take a deep breath in through your nose, extending your ribcage and lungs.
- Slowly exhale via your mouth, thoroughly emptying your lungs.
- Pay attention to how your chest and belly expand and contract with each breath.
- Deep breathing exercises help the body relax and expand the lungs.

Exercises that increase range of motion:

- Move carefully and softly through these exercises to prevent aggravating your joints or muscles.
- Begin with a small number of repetitions and increase them as your flexibility increases.
- Try to be consistent as you incorporate these workouts into your regular regimen.
- Pay attention to your body and avoid forcing yourself into uncomfortable postures; gentle stretches are best.

- Before beginning a new workout plan, speak with a healthcare provider or physical therapist if you have any particular health issues or problems.

CHAPTER SEVEN

LOW IMPACT EXERCISES FOR SPECIFIC HEALTH CONDITIONS

Exercises for Arthritis and Joint Pain

Your quality of life may be greatly impacted by arthritis and joint pain, but regular exercise tailored to your requirements can help you manage pain, increase mobility, and improve your general wellbeing. It's essential to speak with your doctor or a physical therapist before beginning any fitness regimen, particularly if you have arthritis or joint discomfort. They can advise you on the workouts that are best for your situation

1.Low-impact aerobics activities include

walking: Walking is a low-impact activity that strengthens your heart without placing undue strain on your joints. Walk on level surfaces and use supportive footwear.

Swimming: Due to their buoyancy, swimming and water aerobics are low-impact on the joints and provide a full-body exercise. The resistance of the water helps to build muscles without putting undue pressure on joints.

3. Bicycling: The intensity of stationary or recumbent bike riding may be readily changed while being easy on the joints. It increases leg strength and cardiovascular fitness.

2.Range of Motion Exercises:

Joint Circles: To increase joint flexibility, gently rotate your wrists, ankles, knees, and hips.

Finger and Thumb Touches: Extend your fingers, then place a delicate pinching motion with your thumb on each fingertip. This workout enhances joint mobility and finger dexterity.

Neck Mobility: To increase neck mobility, gently move your head to the left and right and tilt it from side to side. Make these motions gently and slowly.

3. **Strength training includes the following:** **Bodyweight Exercises:** To increase muscular strength, carry out bodyweight exercises including squats, modified push-ups, and seated leg lifts. As your strength increases, start with a small number of repetitions and progressively increase.

Resistance bands: To strengthen a range of muscular groups, use resistance bands. Bands are easy on joints and provide resistance without using hefty weights.

Lightweight items: For shoulder presses, tricep extensions, and bicep curls, use light dumbbells or resistance weights. To prevent strain, carry out these exercises with minimal weights and appropriate technique.

4. Stretching and Flexibility Exercise:

Yoga:. Stretching and relaxation-focused gentle yoga postures, in particular, may help increase flexibility and lessen joint stiffness. Look for yoga sessions for beginners or yoga for people in chairs if you have arthritis.

Tai Chi: Tai Chi: Encourages slow, fluid motions that improve equilibrium, flexibility, and joint mobility. Classes often emphasize relaxation methods, which have advantages for both the mind and body.

5. Exercises for balance:

To Stand on One Leg: Lift one foot just a little bit off the ground while holding onto a solid surface. For a few seconds, try to maintain your balance on one leg before switching sides. This exercise develops the leg muscles and enhances stability.

Balance Board Workouts: Using a balancing board tests your equilibrium and develops your stabilizing muscles. Start with easy exercises and advance as your confidence grows.

6. Breathing and relaxation techniques include:

- Practice deep breathing techniques to ease tension and encourage relaxation. Take a big breath in with your nose, hold it for a second, and then gently let it out through your mouth. To unwind your body and mind, pay attention to your breathing.

- Mindfulness and meditation Practice mindfulness or meditation to reduce stress, which may increase the symptoms of arthritis. These techniques enhance mental health and improve your ability to handle pain.

Important Advice:

Warm up before you begin: Always start your workout with a light warm-up to get your muscles and joints ready. Warm packs on the afflicted regions, modest cardiovascular exercise, or joint rotations may all help.

Pay Attention to Your Body: Pay close attention to how your body feels while exercising and afterward. If you feel pain, which should not be mistaken for moderate discomfort, stop what you're doing and talk to your doctor.

Moderation is essential: Start out cautiously, then progressively increase the difficulty and length of your workouts. Joint discomfort might become worse with overexertion.

Keep Hydrated: For lubricated joints, drink lots of water, particularly while working out.

Rest and Recuperation: After workouts, give your body time to relax and repair. Getting enough rest and sleep is essential for controlling arthritic symptoms.

Managing Diabetes through Exercise

By increasing insulin sensitivity, regulating blood sugar levels, and boosting general health, exercise is essential for treating diabetes. People with diabetes may benefit from regular exercise by maintaining a healthy weight, lowering their risk of complications, and living a better quality of life.

1.Consult Your Healthcare Professional: Consult your doctor before beginning any fitness regimen, particularly if you have diabetic difficulties or other health issues. They may provide you individualized advice that is based on your health.

2. Select the Correct Exercise:

- **Exercises for the Heart**: Exercise aerobically via cycling, swimming, dancing, or other means. Aim for 150 minutes or more per week of aerobic activity at a moderate level. Exercises that promote cardiovascular health and blood sugar control are called aerobics.

- **Strengthening Exercises:** Include activities that build strength utilizing bodyweight, weights, or resistance bands. Include strength workouts for the main muscle groups in your regimen, and do them at least twice each week. Increased muscle mass enhances insulin sensitivity and aids in blood sugar control.

- **Flexibility and balancing Exercises:** Incorporate balancing and stretching drills like yoga or Tai Chi. These exercises improve flexibility, balance, and coordination, which lowers the risk of falls and increases mobility in general.

3. Monitor Blood Sugar Levels: Consistently check your blood sugar levels, particularly before and after working out. Monitoring enables you to learn how your body reacts to various workout kinds and make the required corrections.

4. Maintain Your Hydration and Feed Your Body: To keep hydrated during and after exercise, drink lots of water. Additionally, if your blood sugar is low before working out, have a little snack. Afterward, have a healthy lunch or snack to refuel your energy.

5. Practice Safe Exercise:

Warm-Up and Cool-Down: Always begin and conclude your exercise with a warm-up. This encourages a gradual return to rest and helps your body get ready for activity.

Wear Appropriate Shoes: Wear the right shoes if you have diabetic neuropathy to avoid foot damage. Check your feet often for any wounds, blisters, or sores, and get medical attention if necessary.

6. Pay Attention to Your Body: Pay close attention to how your body feels while exercising and afterward. Stop exercising and get medical help if required if you feel faint, out of breath, have chest discomfort, or are very tired.

7. Regular Monitoring and Adaptation: Keep track of your development and modify your training regimen in accordance with your blood sugar levels, general health, and fitness objectives. Make sure your exercise plan complies with your medical requirements by working closely with your healthcare physician and the diabetes care team.

8. Include Lifestyle Changes: A balanced, low-glycemic index diet full of whole grains, fruits, vegetables, lean meats, and healthy fats should be combined with frequent exercise. The advantages of exercise are enhanced by a healthy diet, which also aids in successful blood sugar control.

- **Stress Reduction:** Blood sugar levels may be impacted by ongoing stress. To successfully manage stress, engage in activities that reduce it, such as deep breathing, meditation, or hobbies.
- **Adequate Sleep:** Give sleep first priority since it is essential for maintaining general health and controlling blood sugar. Spend 7-9 hours each night getting a good night's sleep.

9. Maintain Your Consistency: Exercise is an essential part of treating diabetes. Make it a habit to engage in regular physical exercise most days of the week. Over time, even quick, routine exercises like walking may contribute to better health.

Heart-Healthy Exercises for Seniors

Regular physical exercise is crucial for maintaining a healthy heart, particularly as we get older. Exercises that increase cardiovascular fitness, circulation, and general well-being are especially beneficial for seniors.

1. Walking: Walking is a simple workout that anybody can do and has great cardiovascular advantages. Plan to walk for at least 150 minutes per week at a moderate pace. You can walk outside, inside, or on a treadmill. It enhances circulation, expands lung capacity, and fortifies the heart.

2. Aerobic Dancing: Your heart rate may increase, and your cardiovascular endurance can be improved by taking low-impact aerobic dancing courses or practicing dance moves at home. Find senior-specific courses and make sure they emphasize easy motions to prevent joint stress.

3. Swimming and water aerobics: Joint-friendly workouts that offer resistance and improve cardiovascular fitness include swimming and water aerobics. Seniors should use water because of its buoyancy, which lessens stress on joints. Exercise in the water in a nearby pool to strengthen your heart and general endurance.

4. Cycling: While being easy on the joints, riding a stationary or recumbent bike offers great cardiovascular exercise. Decide on a comfortable resistance setting, then cycle slowly. This activity strengthens the legs and strengthens the heart.

5. Exercises for the chair: Seniors who have trouble standing for long periods of time or who have restricted mobility might benefit from chair exercises. While sitting on a sturdy chair, you may increase your heart rate and improve circulation by doing seated leg lifts, seated marches, and seated torso twists.

6. Resistance Band Workouts: Use resistance band workouts to build up different muscle groups. For both upper and lower body exercises, resistance bands provide soft resistance. Muscle development enhances cardiovascular health and promotes mobility in general.

7. Tai Chi: Tai Chi is a low-impact workout that incorporates relaxing breathing exercises and slow, gentle motions. This age-old activity improves flexibility, balance, and cardiovascular fitness. Many localities provide Tai Chi lessons, especially for older citizens.

8. Yoga: Yoga places a strong emphasis on relaxed, regulated breathing and movement. Yoga comes in many different variations, some of which are mild and appropriate for seniors, such as chair yoga or restorative yoga. Yoga enhances mental health, flexibility, and circulation.

9. Balance exercises: These include heel-to-toe walking, standing on one leg, and balance board exercises. Balance exercises test stability and work the core muscles. Enhancing balance lowers the chance of falling and promotes cardiovascular health in general.

10. Mindful Walking and Breathing: Walk mindfully while paying attention to your breath and your body's feelings in a peaceful setting. Deep breathing exercises and slow, deliberate walking may be used to lower stress, quiet the mind, and improve heart health.

Important Things to Keep in Mind

- **Always Warm Up and Cool Down:** Begin with a little warm-up and finish with a cool-down to get your body ready for exercise and encourage relaxation afterward.

- **Pay Attention to Your Body:** Pay close attention to how your body feels while exercising and afterward. Stop the exercise and seek medical attention if you feel pain or discomfort.

- **Stay Hydryated:** Drink water to keep hydrated and help your cardiovascular system before, during, and after exercise.

- **Regular Checkups**: Visit your doctor on a regular basis to assess your heart health and talk about your exercise program to make sure it is in line with your overall health objectives.

CHAPTER EIGHT

INCORPORATING MINDFULNESS AND RELAXATION TECHNIQUES

Breathing Exercises for Stress Reduction

Breathing exercises are powerful tools for reducing stress, calming the mind, and promoting relaxation. They can be practiced anywhere, at any time, and are particularly useful during moments of anxiety or tension. Here are several effective breathing exercises to help you manage stress and cultivate a sense of peace and tranquility:

1. Diaphragmatic Breathing (Deep Belly Breathing):

- Sit or lie down in a comfortable position.
- Place one hand on your chest and the other on your abdomen.
- Inhale deeply through your nose, allowing your diaphragm to expand and your abdomen to rise (your chest should move very little).
- Exhale slowly through your mouth, feeling your abdomen fall.
- Continue this deep breathing pattern for several minutes, focusing on the rise and fall of your abdomen.

2. 4-7-8 Breathing:

- Sit or lie down with your back straight.
- Close your mouth and inhale quietly through your nose to a mental count of four.
- Hold your breath for a count of seven.
- Exhale completely through your mouth to a count of eight.
- This completes one breath cycle. Repeat for a total of four cycles.
- This exercise is calming and can be practiced multiple times a day, especially before bedtime to aid relaxation.

3. Alternate Nostril Breathing (Nadi Shodhana):

- Sit comfortably with your spine straight and shoulders relaxed.
- Use your right thumb to close your right nostril and inhale deeply through your left nostril.
- Close your left nostril with your right ring finger, release your right nostril, and exhale completely.
- Inhale deeply through your right nostril, close it with your right thumb, release your left nostril, and exhale completely.

- This completes one cycle. Repeat for several rounds, focusing on the gentle flow of breath.

4. Box Breathing (Square Breathing):

- Inhale quietly through your nose to a count of four.
- Hold your breath for a count of four.
- Exhale completely through your mouth to a count of four.
- Pause and hold your breath for another count of four.
- Repeat this pattern for several rounds. The square pattern helps balance and calm the mind.

5. Body Scan Breathing:

- Sit or lie down in a comfortable position.
- Close your eyes and bring your attention to your breath.
- As you inhale, imagine your breath traveling through your body, starting from your toes and moving up to your head.
- As you exhale, visualize your breath moving down from your head to your toes.
- With each breath, scan your body for areas of tension and imagine releasing that tension with your exhale.
- Continue this body scan for several minutes, allowing your body to relax and let go of stress.

6. Humming Bee Breathing (Bhramari):

- Sit comfortably with your eyes closed and take a deep breath in.
- Exhale slowly while making a humming sound like a bee, focusing on the vibration in your throat.
- Inhale deeply again and repeat the humming sound on your exhale.
- Feel the calming effect of the humming vibration and continue for several rounds, allowing stress to melt away.

7. Guided Visualization with Breathing:

- Find a quiet and comfortable place to sit or lie down.
- Close your eyes and take a few deep breaths to relax.
- Imagine a peaceful place, such as a beach, forest, or meadow. Visualize the details – the colors, sounds, and smells of that place.
- As you breathe in, imagine you are inhaling the tranquility and calmness of that peaceful place. As you exhale, release any stress or tension.
- Continue breathing deeply and visualizing the serene surroundings, allowing your mind to unwind.

Tips for Effective Breathing Exercises:

Practice Regularly: Consistency is key. Set aside a few minutes each day to practice these breathing exercises, especially during stressful moments.

Create a Quiet Environment: Find a quiet space where you won't be disturbed. You can enhance the atmosphere with calming music, dim lighting, or essential oils.

Be Patient: If your mind starts to wander, gently bring your focus back to your breath. With practice, it becomes easier to maintain concentration.

Combine Breathing with Movement: Consider combining breathing exercises with gentle movements like yoga or stretching for a holistic relaxation experience.

By incorporating these breathing exercises into your routine, you can effectively reduce stress, promote relaxation, and create a sense of calm in your daily life. Remember that these techniques can be customized to fit your preferences, and you can explore different methods to find what works best for you. Regular practice will not only help you manage stress but also enhance your overall well-being.

Meditation and Mindfulness Practices

Meditation and mindfulness are ancient practices that have gained significant popularity in the modern world due to their profound benefits for mental and emotional well-being. These practices involve focusing your mind and eliminating the stream of jumbled thoughts that crowd your consciousness, ultimately leading to a sense of clarity, tranquility, and enhanced self-awareness. Here's how you can begin your journey into meditation and mindfulness:

1. Mindful Breathing Meditation:

- Find a quiet and comfortable place to sit or lie down.
- Close your eyes and bring your attention to your breath. Notice the sensation of your breath entering and leaving your body.
- Breathe naturally and focus on the rise and fall of your chest or the sensation of the breath passing through your nostrils.
- Whenever your mind starts to wander (as it naturally will), gently guide your focus back to your breath.
- Start with a few minutes and gradually increase the duration as you become more comfortable.

2. Body Scan Meditation:

- Lie down in a comfortable position, arms at your sides and palms facing up.
- Close your eyes and bring your awareness to your toes. Feel any sensations in your toes without judgment.
- Slowly move your focus to each part of your body, paying attention to any tension, sensations, or areas of relaxation.
- Allow yourself to release any tension you notice. This practice promotes relaxation and body awareness.

3. Loving-Kindness Meditation (Metta):

- Sit in a comfortable position with your eyes closed.
- Begin by generating feelings of love and compassion for yourself. Repeat phrases like, "May I be happy, may I be healthy, may I live with ease."
- Extend these feelings to others, starting with someone you care about deeply. Repeat the phrases for them: "May you be happy, may you be healthy, may you live with ease."
- Gradually extend these feelings to acquaintances, strangers, and even people you have conflicts with. Cultivate feelings of love and kindness for all beings.

4. Guided Meditation:

- Use guided meditation recordings or apps that lead you through a meditation practice. These can focus on relaxation, gratitude, self-compassion, or any other topic.
- Find a quiet space, put on headphones, and follow the guidance of the meditation instructor.
- Guided meditations are excellent for beginners, as they provide structure and support during the practice.

5. Walking Meditation:

- Find a peaceful and quiet place to walk, either indoors or outdoors.
- As you walk, focus your attention on the sensation of walking. Feel your feet lifting, moving through the air, and making contact with the ground.
- Pay attention to each step and the movements of your body. Engage all your senses in the experience of walking.
- Walking meditation can be a wonderful way to combine mindfulness with physical activity.

6. Mindful Eating:

- Choose a small piece of food, such as a raisin or a nut.

- Examine the food item with curiosity, noticing its texture, color, and shape.

- Smell the food, paying attention to its aroma.

- Take a small bite and chew slowly, noticing the taste and texture. Be fully present in the experience of eating.

- This practice encourages mindfulness and gratitude for the nourishment provided by food.

7. Mindfulness in Daily Activities:

- Bring mindfulness to everyday tasks such as washing dishes, showering, or walking the dog.

- Focus on the sensations, sounds, and movements associated with the activity.

- Be fully present in the moment, appreciating the simple aspects of life that are often taken for granted.

- Cultivate a sense of mindfulness throughout your day, anchoring yourself in the present moment.

Tips for Practicing Meditation and Mindfulness:

Consistency is Key: Regular practice, even for a few minutes each day, yields the most significant benefits. Establish a daily routine for your meditation and mindfulness practices.

Non-Judgmental Awareness: Approach your thoughts and feelings with gentle curiosity and non-judgment. Mindfulness is about observing without criticism.

Be Patient: It's natural for your mind to wander during meditation. When you notice your mind has drifted, gently bring your focus back to the present moment.

Create a Comfortable Environment: Find a quiet and comfortable space where you won't be disturbed. Dim lighting and soft music, if desired, can enhance your meditation experience.

Openness to Learning: Explore different meditation and mindfulness techniques to find what resonates with you. There are various styles, so experiment and find the practices that bring you the most peace and relaxation.

The Importance of Adequate Sleep for Seniors

Adequate sleep is crucial for people of all ages, but it holds particular significance for seniors. Quality sleep plays a fundamental role in maintaining good physical and mental health, supporting cognitive function, and promoting emotional well-being. Here's why sufficient sleep is essential for seniors and how it contributes to their overall quality of life:

1. Physical Health:

Immune Function: Quality sleep strengthens the immune system, helping the body fend off infections and illnesses. Seniors with adequate sleep are better equipped to fight off diseases.

Heart Health: Proper sleep contributes to a healthy heart. It regulates blood pressure, reduces the risk of heart diseases, and supports overall cardiovascular health.

Weight Management: Lack of sleep disrupts hormones that regulate hunger and appetite, often leading to weight gain. Seniors who sleep well are better able to maintain a healthy weight.

Pain Management: Sleep plays a role in pain modulation. Adequate rest can reduce pain sensitivity and improve seniors' ability to manage chronic pain conditions.

2. Cognitive Function:

Memory and Learning: During sleep, the brain processes and consolidates memories from the day. Seniors who sleep well have improved memory retention and learning abilities.

Brain Health: Sufficient sleep supports brain health and reduces the risk of cognitive decline and neurodegenerative diseases, such as Alzheimer's and dementia.

Problem-Solving Skills: A well-rested brain is more adept at problem-solving, decision-making, and maintaining mental clarity.

3. Emotional Well-Being:

Mood Regulation: Lack of sleep can lead to irritability, anxiety, and mood swings. Seniors who sleep well are more emotionally resilient and better able to cope with stress.

Reduced Risk of Depression: Adequate sleep is associated with a reduced risk of depression and helps in managing symptoms for seniors already experiencing depressive disorders.

Emotional Balance: Quality sleep contributes to emotional balance and helps seniors maintain a positive outlook on life.

4. Balance and Fall Prevention:

Balance and Coordination: Sufficient sleep enhances balance and coordination, reducing the risk of falls and related injuries. Seniors who sleep well are steadier on their feet.

Fall Prevention: Lack of sleep can lead to dizziness and impaired reflexes, increasing the risk of falls. Adequate rest improves seniors' ability to navigate their environment safely.

5. Social and Interpersonal Relationships:

Improved Communication: Seniors who are well-rested can engage in conversations more effectively. Adequate sleep enhances communication skills and active listening abilities.

Enhanced Social Interactions: Seniors who sleep well are more likely to engage in social activities, fostering meaningful connections with friends, family, and the community.

6. Quality of Life:

Overall Well-Being: Adequate sleep significantly contributes to an improved quality of life for seniors. It ensures they wake up feeling refreshed and ready to face the day, leading to a more positive and fulfilling life experience.

Longevity: Studies suggest that regular, restorative sleep can contribute to a longer lifespan, emphasizing the importance of healthy sleep patterns for seniors.

Tips for Seniors to Improve Sleep Quality:

Establish a Sleep Routine: Maintain a consistent sleep schedule, going to bed and waking up at the same time every day, even on weekends.

Create a Relaxing Bedtime Routine: Engage in calming activities before bedtime, such as reading, gentle stretching, or listening to soothing music.

Optimize Sleep Environment: Make your bedroom comfortable, dark, quiet, and cool. Invest in a supportive mattress and pillows.

Limit Stimulants: Avoid caffeine and nicotine close to bedtime, as these substances can interfere with sleep.

Stay Active: Engage in regular physical activity, but avoid vigorous exercise close to bedtime.

Limit Naps: If napping during the day affects your ability to sleep at night, consider limiting daytime naps.

CONCLUSION

In the journey toward healthy aging, embracing holistic well-being is paramount. Our discussion has highlighted various facets of senior health, from low-impact exercises tailored for older adults to the significance of meditation, mindfulness practices, and the essential role of adequate sleep. By integrating these elements into their lives, seniors can enjoy not only physical vitality but also mental acuity, emotional resilience, and an enhanced quality of life.

Physical Health Through Gentle Exercise:

Engaging in low-impact exercises, such as walking, swimming, or chair-based workouts, fosters physical strength, flexibility, and cardiovascular health. These exercises, when performed regularly, aid in maintaining a healthy weight, managing chronic conditions, and preventing falls, ensuring seniors can lead active and independent lives.

Mindfulness and Meditation:

The practice of mindfulness and meditation offers seniors a gateway to tranquility and emotional balance. By cultivating present-moment awareness, seniors can reduce stress, improve cognitive function, and foster a positive outlook on life. These practices provide essential tools for managing challenges, enhancing resilience, and nurturing a deep sense of inner peace.

The Vital Role of Adequate Sleep:

Adequate sleep is foundational to overall well-being. Seniors who prioritize sleep benefit from strengthened immunity, improved memory, emotional stability, and reduced risks of chronic illnesses. Quality sleep not only supports physical health but also rejuvenates the mind, enhancing cognitive abilities and promoting emotional resilience.

Incorporating these practices into daily life fosters a harmonious balance between physical, mental, and emotional health. However, it's crucial to approach these practices with patience and consistency, adapting them to individual needs and preferences. Moreover, consulting healthcare professionals ensures a tailored approach, addressing specific health concerns and maximizing the benefits of these holistic practices.

As seniors embrace these principles of holistic well-being, they embark on a transformative journey toward a fulfilling and vibrant senior hood. By nourishing their bodies, minds, and spirits, seniors empower themselves to savor life's moments, maintain meaningful relationships, and cultivate a deep sense of contentment. Through these practices, the senior years can truly become a golden chapter marked by vitality, serenity, and a profound sense of well-being.

www.ingramcontent.com/pod-product-compliance
Lightning Source LLC
Chambersburg PA
CBHW050830260726

48660CB00006B/2162